I0706642

Get Rid of Cellulite for Good.

A Nutritionist's Guide – How Eating the Right Foods Can Help You Fight Cellulite and Banish It for Good.

By Laura Hails.

Contents

3

Introduction

The food we eat creates the person that we become, eat healthy, nutritious food and you will look radiant, have more energy, sleep more soundly, become more active, lose excess weight and ultimately, achieve more.

There is no miracle cure for cellulite, there are no overnight solutions, magic creams or potions but there is a solution and that solution lies with your diet. Simply put, eat the right diet combined with the right exercise plan and the results can be dramatic.

Scientific studies have proved that by combining the right foods in our diet with a fitness regime that builds muscle as well as burning calories then the appearance of cellulite can be dramatically reduced.

This book will explain what a nutritious diet should look like, tips on how to introduce a healthy diet into your life and the foods that you should be consuming more of to help you lose the pounds and lose the cellulite.

Chapter One

Cellulite Explained

What is cellulite

Cellulite is comprised of fat and fluids trapped in pockets of connective tissue beneath the service of the skin which causes the cells to pucker. The thin layer of connective tissue between fat cells starts to thicken and pull together around the fat, causing tiny dimples and irregularities characteristic with cellulite. The fat inside the cells bulges out and the more fat you have the worse the bulging.

What causes cellulite

Cellulite is essentially the result of too much fat and too little muscle. When the underlying muscle becomes too thin and the overlying fat becomes too thick, there is no firm base for the skin, which then takes on the wobbly, irregular appearance we call cellulite.

Failing to do enough exercise has serious consequences. Without regular toning exercise you start to lose muscle after the age of 20. Between the ages of 20 and 30 years the average non-exercise woman loses 5lb of muscle, a further 5lb between the ages of 30 and 40 and a similar amount each decade after that. The result is a loss of strength as well as increase in fat storage.

As you lose muscle, your metabolic rate drops. Muscle burns calories, so the less you have the fewer calories you need. So, as you get older you need fewer calories just to maintain your body weight. For every 5lbs loss of muscle, your metabolic rate drops by 5%.

Age related muscle loss means that you burn fewer calories and store more of them as fat. Even if you continue eating the same amount of food and keeping the same lifestyle, your weight will increase as your body converts the excess calories into stored fat.

For most women this extra fat is stored around the hips and thighs. When an area has too much fat, too little muscle and weak connective tissue, it loses its normal firm appearance and takes on the characteristic wobbly appearance associated with cellulite.

How to fight cellulite

Getting rid of cellulite is not easy and cannot be done overnight. Whilst there are many claims of cellulite cures ranging from diets and pills to creams and treatments scientific studies have shown that the most effective way to get rid of cellulite is a combination of the right diet and the right exercise.

Reducing your calorie intake whilst increasing your daily calorie burn creates a calorie deficit so your body has no choice but to use up its fat stores.

Diet Guidelines

1 - Eat five or more portions of fruit and vegetables each day

2 - Avoid saturated and processed fats

3 - Eat foods high in fibre and water

4 - Include wholegrains and cereals in your daily diet

5 - Eat more beans and lentils

6 - Eat nuts and seeds regularly

7 - Drink 2 litres of water a day

8 - Avoid refined sugars and flour.

Exercise

The key is to include both strength (toning) training to build muscle as well as cardiovascular (aerobic) exercise to burn fat in your exercise programme. Strength training doesn't necessarily mean lifting heavy weights. It can be toning exercises using your own body weight, light hand-held weights, exercise bands or tubes for resistance.

Don't be afraid of adding strength exercises, as your muscles tone up, they'll become firmer and smaller. As you get older collagen and elastin fibres become less elastic which makes your fat more noticeable. But as you build muscle, the fibres are strengthened, reducing dimples, so the appearance of your cellulite will dramatically improve.

More muscle means more calories burned during activity as well as when resting. Every 1lb of muscle you add through exercise increases your metabolic rate by 30 – 40 calories a day.

Chapter Two
Small Changes

Making small changes can have big results. There are hundreds of foods that you can add to your diet that will help you lose weight and fight cellulite. Try to build good habits into your daily regime and over time you will reap the rewards.

Breakfast –

Make time for breakfast, studies show that people that skip breakfast are more likely to overeat later in the day. Try to eat a high protein breakfast that will keep you fuller for longer.

People who start their day with a healthy filling breakfast dramatically increase their chances of eating healthily throughout the day. People who eat a good, breakfast feel more satisfied and energized for the rest of the day.

No time for breakfast – blitz up a smoothie, add bananas and berries with a spoonful of live bio yoghurt and a splash of milk or fruit juice.

Avoid temptation.

Lunch –

Pack your own lunch, that way you will control the calories you are consuming, and you won't be tempted with the bakery. People who eat out consume 300 calories more than those who pack their own lunch.

Eating a low-fat salad or fruit can cut your calories by up to 12%. Salad and fruit contain a lot of water, which means you eat less of the higher calorie foods.

Start your meal with soup. The fibre in soup fills you up which means you are less likely to eat higher calorie foods afterwards. Drinking soup at lunch time can reduce your calorie intake by up to 20%.

Make your lunchtime sandwich healthier by opting for pitta bread or wholegrain. Fill it with lots of salad, hummus and avocado.

Dinner –

Go easy on the pasta and potatoes in your evening meal and opt for more vegetables, salad and lean protein instead. If you must eat carbs in the evening a good guideline is to ensure that you don't eat any more than 2oz (dried weight) of pasta or rice and 5oz of potatoes. Swap potatoes for sweet potatoes, sweet potatoes release energy slower and therefore keep you feeling fuller for longer.

Chapter Three

A Nutritional Diet

<u>Proteins</u>

Protein is a powerful nutrient, it plays a major role in our body, building body tissue and making important hormones. Proteins are made up of a collection of 20 amino acids, these are divided into two - "essential" which are sourced from your food and "non-essential that are produced by your body.

Protein, will keep you fuller for longer, it will help you concentrate, reduce sugar cravings, give you energy and keep your hair, nails and bones strong. The protein in your body is constantly being broken down and replaced. The body does not store amino acids like it does carbohydrates and fats, so it needs a daily supply of amino acids to make new proteins. The protein in the food you eat is digested into amino acids that can be used to replace the protein in your body.

There are two different types of proteins in our diet, complete and incomplete. The difference between the two is determined by its amino acid composition.

Complete Proteins – These are proteins that supply all "essential amino acids" complete proteins come from foods such as eggs, milk, meat, fish and soy.

Complete proteins are great sauces of protein and should make up 75% of our daily protein intake, however you can combine incomplete proteins with complete proteins to ensure you are getting the complete range of "essential amino acids" in your diet.

Animal Derived Complete Proteins – Meat, poultry, fish and shellfish all contain all the "essential" amino acids. Fish and shellfish are a particularly good source of complete protein because they are low fat and rich in essential minerals. Examples include shrimp, scallops, clams, tuna, salmon, mackerel, halibut, sardines and cod.

Vegetarian, Animal Derived Complete Proteins – Eggs and dairy products are also complete proteins, containing all essential amino acids. Examples are eggs, cheese and yoghurt. Quorn – although not derived from animals is a plant based complete protein but as it contains some dairy it cannot be classed as vegan.

Vegan, Plant Based Complete Proteins - Plant-based foods that are complete protein choices, include soy products, quinoa and buckwheat – which are a protein-rich whole grain. Soybeans form the basis of many processed soy foods, all of which are complete protein sources, such as soy milk, tempeh, tofu, miso and edamame which are fresh green soybeans.

Incomplete Proteins – These are proteins that do not contain all essential amino acids, or don't have sufficient quantities of them to meet the body's needs and should be combined with other proteins. Examples of incomplete proteins are nuts and seeds, pulses, grains such as rice and vegetables.

These proteins shouldn't be ignored as they contribute towards a healthy, balanced diet. Proteins that in combination with each other provide the complete range of essential amino acids are called complementary proteins. Complimentary proteins don't have to be combined at the same meal, but they should be combined within the same day as the body does not store the protein it consumes.

Examples of complementary proteins are – rice and beans, spinach and almonds, hummus and whole grain pittas.

<u>Carbohydrates –</u>

Dietary carbohydrates are split into three categories:

Sugars – these are short chain carbohydrates that are found in foods, examples of sugar carbohydrates are glucose,

Starches – these are long chains of glucose molecules, which eventually get broken down into glucose in the digestive system these are found in potatoes, corn and oats, peas and rice.

Fibre – Humans cannot digest fibre, but the bacteria in the digestive system can make use of some of them, fibre is essential for a healthy digestive system. Fibre is found in vegetables, fruit, salad, pulses and whole grains.

The most important thing to know about carbohydrates is that you need them to give you energy, by eating the right foods you naturally become more energetic, you do more, and you burn off more calories. A balanced diet helps with weight control, sleeping patterns and memory and concentration levels. The key is to eat the right carbs and ditch the wrong ones

Carbohydrates in their natural form are good for you and should be part of a healthy, balanced diet. Whilst cutting down on simple carbohydrates such as biscuits, cakes and pastries will increase your wellbeing and help you maintain a healthy diet you shouldn't be tempted to cut complex carbohydrates from your diet.

Carbohydrates are not essential as the body can function without them, however, complex carbohydrates are an important part of a healthy diet because of their high nutritional value. Cut back on simple carbohydrates and increase the complex ones.

The More Complex the better

Complex Carbs are starch and fibre and have more nutrients then Simple Carbs. They have a higher fibre content and therefore, digest more slowly making you feel fuller for longer.

Complex carbohydrates are more filling and therefore will help you control your weight, they also help keep your blood sugars level, which stops cravings.

Complex Carbohydrates you should be eating –

fruit, vegetables, nuts, pulses and whole grains, whole wheat bread and cereal, corn, oats, peas and brown or wild rice.

1 - whole grains – these are good sources of fibre, as well as potassium, magnesium and selenium. Choose - quinoa, buckwheat, and whole – wheat pasta and noodles

2 - Fruit – such as apples, berries and bananas.

3 - Vegetables – all vegetables, but in particular, leafy greens such as spinach, kale and cabbage.

4 - Beans – beans, peas and lentils.

Fats –

Good fats – Oil rich, nutritious foods like <u>nuts, seeds and avocados</u> are rich in omega 3 and 6 fatty acids which protect against heart disease, aid weight loss, lower cholesterol and promote healthy hair, nails and skin. Another way to get essential fat is to use <u>cold pressed oils such as rapeseed, extra virgin olive oil, walnut and sesame oil.</u>

Chapter Four

Eat the Rainbow

Antioxidants

Antioxidants come up frequently in discussions about good health and preventing diseases. These powerful substances, which mostly come from the fresh fruits and vegetables we eat, prohibit (and in some cases even prevent), the oxidation of other molecules in the body. The benefits of antioxidants are very important to good health, because if free radicals are left unchallenged, they can cause a wide range of illnesses and chronic diseases.

Antioxidants and Free Radicals

The human body naturally produces free radicals and the

antioxidants to counteract their damaging effects. However, in most cases, free radicals far outnumber the naturally occurring antioxidants. In order to maintain the balance, and maximise

the benefits of antioxidants a continual supply of external sources of antioxidants are necessary. Antioxidants benefit the body by neutralising and removing the free radicals from the bloodstream.

Different Antioxidants Benefit Different Parts of the Body

There are a wide range of antioxidants found in nature, and because they are so varied, different antioxidants provide benefits to different parts of the body. For example, beta-carotene (and other carotenoids) is very beneficial for healthy eyes, lycopene is beneficial for helping maintain prostate health; flavonoids are especially beneficial in maintaining a healthy heart; and proanthocyanins are beneficial for urinary tract health.

Antioxidants and Skin Health Benefits

When skin is exposed to high levels of ultraviolet light, photooxidative damage is induced by the formation of different types of reactive species of oxygen, including singlet oxygen, superoxide radicals, and peroxide radicals. These forms of reactive oxygen damage cellular lipids, proteins, and DNA, and they are considered to be the primary contributors to erythema (sunburn), premature aging of the skin, photo dermatoses, and skin cancers.

Antioxidants and Immune System Support

Singlet oxygen can compromise the immune system, because it has the ability to catalyze production of free radicals. Astaxanthin and Spirulina have been shown to enhance both the non-specific and specific immune system, and to protect cell membranes and cellular DNA from mutation. Astaxanthin is the single most powerful quencher of singlet oxygen, and is up to ten times stronger than other carotenoids (including beta-carotene), and up to 500 times stronger than alpha tocopherol (Vitamin E), while Spirulina has a variety of antioxidants and other substances that are beneficial in boosting immunity.

Additional Ways Antioxidants Help Benefit our Health

Increasing one's antioxidant intake is essential for optimum health, especially in today's polluted world. Because the body just can't keep up with antioxidant production, a good amount of these vitamins, minerals, phytochemicals, and enzymes must come from our daily diet. Boosting your antioxidant intake can help provide added protection for the body against heart problems, eye problems, memory problems, mood disorders and immune system problems.

Top Antioxidant – rich Fruit and Vegetables.

Blackberries, blueberries, broccoli, Brussel sprouts, Curly kale, garlic, plums, prunes, raisins, raspberries, red peppers, spinach and strawberries.

Plant Nutrients -

The more variety and colour you eat the more nutrients you will consume and the more benefit you will get from your diet.

According to a recent National Diet and Nutrition Survey many of our diets - adults and children - are lacking in vitamin A and

D, selenium and zinc and many women are lacking calcium and iron.

Fruit and vegetables are considered so good for us that nutritionists suggest that the recommended government 5 a day should be our bare minimum. But the truth is that most people aren't even eating 5 a day. Fruit and vegetables provide a huge variety of vitamins, minerals and fibre and if you are missing out on eating them you will leave a big gap in the nutrients you consume.

The best way to get the most from your food is variety. Many people get stuck in a rut, eating the same food day in and day out with little or no variety. In order to stay healthy, the body needs over 40 different vitamins and minerals a day so sticking to the same foods will hugely reduce your intake.

Introducing new and different foods to your weekly shop will not only keep your food exciting but your body will reap the rewards.

Whilst some foods have significant health benefits it is important to remember that no one individual food can treat, prevent or cure health problems, the key is to eat all foods as part of a balanced diet.

Include fruit and vegetables from the five colour groups, red, orange, yellow, green and purple. Different coloured fruit and vegetables contain different nutrients, combining them is the best way to ensure you get all you need.

Many of the naturally occurring chemicals responsible for giving fruit and veg their bright colours actually help keep us healthy and free from disease. Fruit and vegetables contain hundreds of colourful phytochemicals that act as antioxidants.

Antioxidant-rich fruit and vegetables can help to protect against heart disease, cancer, and premature aging.

Red–

Many red foods contain high levels of vitamin C. They contain high levels of anthocyanins which are linked to being effective in fighting cancer, bacterial infections and neurological diseases.

Red fruit and vegetables to include in your diet

are raspberries, cranberries, strawberries, cherries, pomegranate, apples, rhubarb, red peppers, tomatoes and watermelon.

Orange

Orange fruit and vegetables are high in carotenoids, crucial for maintaining a good immune system and supporting cell repair and healthy vision.

Orange fruit and vegetables to include in your diet are Carrots, oranges, squashes, sweet potatoes, mangoes, peaches, nectarines, pumpkins, swede and peppers.

Yellow

Yellow fruit and vegetables contain large amounts of bioflavonoids, which fight infection and reduce inflammation.

Yellow fruit and vegetables to introduce into your diet – corn, pineapple, peppers and squashes.

Green

Green fruit and vegetables contain nutrients including lutein, lycopene, folic acid, zeaxanthin and glycosylates all of which are associated with helping to prevent cancer.

Green fruit and vegetables to include in your diet

- asparagus, avocado, rocket, spinach, lettuce, watercress, cucumber, broccoli, Brussels sprouts, leafy cabbage, spring greens, beans, peas, sugar snap peas, mange tout, cress, courgette, peppers, spring onions, leeks, apples, grapes and kiwi fruit.

Purple/blue

Purple and blue fruit and vegetables are high in antioxidants which promote healthy blood and are believed to have antiaging properties.

Purple and blue fruit and vegetables to include in your diet are blackberries, blueberries, grapes, blackcurrants, plums, red cabbage, prunes, red onions, olives, purple sprouting broccoli, beetroot and aubergine.

Chapter Five

A Balanced Plate

Eat more than just the rainbow - As well as a variety of fruit, salad and vegetables we should also be eating beans, fish, nuts and seeds and good oils.

Beans –

Also known as pulses or legumes, pulses are packed with complete protein and contain almost no fat and are a good source of complex carbohydrates which are essential for good health.

Studies have linked that a higher consumption of beans results in a lower risk of heart disease and developing type 2 diabetes. It is now believed that a good intake of beans probably reduces the risk of stomach and prostate cancer.

Beans are low in fat and saturates and are packed with

insoluble and soluble fibre, protein and a variety of minerals. Insoluble fibre helps keep our digestive system healthy whilst soluble fibre helps to control blood sugar levels and lowers cholesterol which means a lower risk of heart disease.

Beans provide potassium a nutrient that helps maintain fluid balance and helps to lower blood pressure. They also contain magnesium and phosphorus which strengthen bones. Many beans contain copper which gives us healthy skin and hair as well as a healthy immune system heart. Most beans provide manganese which is important for brain function and the metabolism of carbs and fat.

Beans are high in protein as well as good source of iron which makes them perfect for vegetarians and vegans. Because they contain both protein and fibre they keep us feeling fuller for longer. They help to slow down the absorption of sugar into the blood which means sugar levels stay even, this is not only good news for people trying to lose weight as it controls the appetite but also good news for people with type 2 diabetes who need to prevent dramatic rises in blood sugar.

Choose from - Aduki beans, black eyed beans, borlotti beans, chickpeas, fava beans, haricot beans, kidney beans, lentils, mung beans, soybeans and split peas.

Nuts –

There are many health benefits to eating nuts, they help lower your cholesterol, lower blood pressure and help you lose weight. The high fat content in nuts make them good for your heart because they are rich in polyunsaturated and monounsaturated fats which lower cholesterol.

Almonds – contain the most fibre, calcium and vitamin B2 which are good for healthy bones, skin, eyesight, red blood cells, nervous system and digestive system.

Brazil Nuts – have a very high selenium content, which is an antioxidant that is essential for a healthy immune system and protects against disease causing free radical damage.

Cashew Nuts – contain the most iron and make them a brilliant choice for vegetarians. Eat with vitamin C rich foods or a glass of orange juice to help the body absorb the iron more easily.

Peanuts – contain the least amount of calories and fat but the most amount of protein and B vitamins. Studies have also shown that people who ate a handful of peanuts twice a week significantly reduced their risk of bowel cancer.

Pistachios – has one of the lowest calories and fat content of other nuts and are the only nut to contain an antioxidant called lutein. Lutein is found in green vegetables and is good for healthy eyes.

Walnuts – are a great source of omega 3, walnuts contain alpha- linolenic acid which the body uses to make omega 3 fats that are found in oily fish such as salmon and mackerel.

Seeds –

Seeds are high in fats that are good for the heart as well as containing beneficial vitamins such as A, B, C, and E and nutrients such as iron, potassium, magnesium, phosphorus, copper, zinc and manganese. Just 30g of pumpkin seeds contain six times more iron then a small roasted chicken and 15% more than a small grilled rump steak, which makes them brilliant for vegetarians and vegans.

Sunflower seeds, flax seeds, alfalfa seeds, pumpkin seeds and sesame seeds are particularly beneficial. Seeds are so nutrient-dense that you don't have to eat a lot of them. Use them in cooking as garnishes or to flavour stews and casseroles, sprinkle them on soup, salads and roasted vegetables. Add them to cereals or smoothies or eat them as a snack.

Grains –

Grains are rich in nutrients and are basic energy foods. Almost all whole, unrefined grains can be beneficial to your health, generally the darker the colour the healthier it is.

Barley – pot barley is the wholegrain version. Barley is good for digestion. It is low in gluten.

Brown Rice – is beneficial for the nervous system and digestive system. It is the least allergenic of all grains. Basmati is perfect for people are overweight.

Buckwheat – is gluten free and rich in healthy minerals. A perfect choice for people who are sensitive to wheat. It is a good source of protein.

Millet – is high in iron, magnesium, potassium, the B vitamins and vitamin E. Millet helps to support the digestive system, improves nutrient uptake and is a great energy booster.

Quinoa – comes from South America. It contains all the essential amino acids and is therefore a complete protein but is easier to digest than meat protein and contains less fat.

Oats – contain more good fats then other grains. They are also a good source of vitamin B Complex which is good for the nervous system and for strengthening bones.

Spelt – like buckwheat is packed with minerals and protein. It is a good alternative for people who are sensitive to wheat, it helps stimulate the immune system and provides a good source of constant energy.

Fish –

Eating more fish is an important part of a healthy diet. Fish is a good source of protein. White fish and shellfish are low in fat and therefore low in calories. Studies have linked good intakes

of fish with a reduced risk of heart disease, depression, dementia and Alzheimer's disease. There is evidence that eating more fish may even reduce the risk of certain cancers.

<u>White Fish</u> – have a significant amount of B vitamins. White fish also contains iodine and selenium, nutrients that are essential for a healthy immune system.

Plaice – is particularly high in biotin which is needed for healthy hair and nails.

Sea Bream – is good for boosting vitamin B6 which is needed for making red blood cells.

Halibut – is one of the best sources of vitamin B3 which is essential for a healthy nervous system and releases energy from food.

Lemon sole and haddock – are good sources of iodine.

<u>Oil Rich Fish</u> – are packed with omega 3 fats which help prevent heart disease, heart attacks and strokes. Omega 3 fats are important for brain cell development particularly before babies are born and in the first few years of childhood.

Oily fish are also rich in vitamin D a nutrient that helps the body absorb calcium which keeps bones strong.

Sardines – not only contain calcium but also high levels of vitamin D.

Tuna (fresh not tinned) – contains high levels of selenium and iron which is an important nutrient for healthy blood.

Salmon – contains good amounts of omega 3 fats as well as being a particularly good source of vitamin E and vitamin B6.

Mackerel – contains one of the richest sources of omega 3 fats as well as iodine and vitamin D.

<u>Shellfish</u> – provide zinc which is essential for normal growth, enzyme function, wound healing, fertility and a healthy immune system.

Scallops – are particularly nutritious, they contain more selenium than either white fish or oily fish and tend to have more iron.

Muscles – are also a good source of iron.

Crab – is a good source of copper which is an important mineral for healthy hear and skin as well as a healthy immune and nervous system.

Prawns – have a higher cholesterol content then other fish but the cholesterol levels in prawns has little effect on blood cholesterol in the body and it is far more important to cut down on saturated fats.

Good Oils –

There are many different types of oils on the market, choosing the right one will bring nutritional value to your cooking.

On the whole oils contain less saturated fat then animal fats such as butter and lard. And more polyunsaturated and monounsaturated fats which can lower your cholesterol.

Cooking oils which are liquid when kept at room temperature are mostly derived from plants, nuts and seeds. They all have a similar amount of calories, which is approx. 100kcal per 1 tbsp. but they differ in the type of fat they contain and their smoke point, which is the temperature at which they start to break down. When the smoke point is reached, the quality, flavour and nutritional benefits are affected. It is important to understand what oils are best for what type of use.

Ground Nut Oil – is made from peanuts and is wonderful for your heart. It is packed with plant sterols that can lower your risk of heart disease. Ground nut oil – as its name would suggest – has a slightly nutty but mild flavour and is very versatile. It has a high smoke point which makes it a good oil to use for grilling or frying.

Olive Oil – is rich in monounsaturated fats which boost good cholesterol and have a beneficial effect on your heart. Olive oil can be heated to higher temperatures which makes it perfect for grilling, baking, roasting or stirring through pastas.

Light Olive Oil – means that the oil is lighter in colour and flavour and it has a higher smoke point making it good for grilling and frying. The term "light" does not mean that it contains fewer calories or fat content.

Extra Virgin Olive Oil – is richer in antioxidants. It has a lower smoke point which means that it loses much of its nutritional benefits when heated. Use it for dressing and sauces that don't need to be cooked.

Rapeseed Oil – is a good all-rounder. Low in saturated fats and high in heart friendly monounsaturated fats rapeseed oil also contains omega 3 and vitamin E. This oil is great in salad dressings but also, because it has a high smoke point it is also perfect for frying, roasting and baking.

Sunflower Oil – is low in saturated fats, rich in polyunsaturated fat – omega 6, and vitamin E. It is a good all-purpose oil, its mild flavour makes it good for using in salads and dressings and its high smoke point means it is also good for frying, roasting and grilling.

Toasted Sesame Oil – is most associated with oriental dishes because of its rich, nutty flavour. It is a good sauce of oleic acid which is good for the heart. Its low smoke point means it is not good for cooking – unless you combine it with another oil, such as Olive or Sunflower oil. It is best used for its flavour in salad dressings or dips.

Chapter Six

Rules for Healthy Living.

Cook from scratch

Take responsibility for what you are eating by knowing exactly what is in your food. Cooking from scratch doesn't have to be complicated or time consuming. look for quick, simple recipes, the fewer the ingredients the quicker the dish, and use good quality ingredients to maximise nutrition. Plan ahead and know what you are going to cook and adapt your menu to the time you have. The recipes in this plan will help you do just that.

Read the labels

Food labels are a reliable, accurate source of valuable nutritional information. Use the labels on the foods you buy to ensure that you are consuming what you think you are consuming. Ingredients are listed in descending order by weight and include any colour, additives, preservatives and, nutrients, fats or sugar that have been added to the product. Whatever appears first on the list is the largest ingredient. Foods with high levels of sugar, salt or saturated fats at the top of the list should be avoided.

Know your Sugar

Sugar comes in many forms with many different names, but it is all the same and has the same effect on the body. Products with sugar listed at the top of its ingredients list is more than likely high in sugar. The following are all sugars – brown sugar, cane juice lactose, maltose, raw cane sugar, raw sugar, sucrose sugar, invert sugar, glucose, fructose, dextrose, corn syrup, corn sweetener.

Consider naturally sweet alternatives such as raw honey or maple syrup or add fruit such as apples, apricots and berries. Carrot or apple juice makes a great base for vegetable juices as they add sweetness.

Know Your Fats

Good fats or "essential fatty acids" as they are known come from nuts and seeds, fish and avocados, they are important for a healthy, balanced diet. These can also be added to your cooking by using them as oils such as sunflower and pumpkin seed oil, macadamia, coconut, walnut, hazelnut and olive oils are all beneficial fats that support nerve function, mental alertness, concentration and memory.

Bad fats or saturated / trans fats are known to raise levels of cholesterol and increase the risk of heart disease. These are found mainly in animal produce and dairy products they are in butter, lard, margarine, cooking fats, chocolate, biscuits, cakes, savory snacks and processed foods.

Read the label and avoid anything that says it contains "hydrogenated" or "partially hydrogenated oils"

Add colour

The more colour in your diet the more goodness you will consume. Each colour of fruit and vegetables contains different and important antioxidants. Antioxidants are part of a well- balanced, healthy diet, they will keep you well throughout the winter months by helping your immune system to kill harmful bacteria and infections and they will keep your skin and hair looking good and give you vitality. Vitamins A, C and E are all found in fresh fruit and vegetables and are all antioxidants.

Be prepared

Always make a meal plan and a shopping list before shopping.
Consider the week ahead in advance. Think about foods that
you love and how you can introduce more variety to them.
Don't be afraid to find recipes and tweak them to suit your own
tastes you may discover something wonderful.

Consider days that you might be home late or have more work
to do than normal and make those evening meals simple and
quick or even prepare them at the weekend, or when you have
more time, and freeze them so that they are at hand when you
need a quick meal. Making your own microwave meals
doesn't need to be either complicated or time consuming – it
just needs planning. Consider, omelets, stir fries or salads with
fresh or tinned fish.

Stay Hydrated

Dehydration can, falsely, make you think that you are hungry.
Your brain can confuse thirst with hunger. Before reaching for
a biscuit or sweets make a conscious effort to have a glass of
water and then decide whether you were hungry or thirsty. If
you really are hungry consider what you are reaching for.

Healthy Snacking.

Snacking between meals is a good thing. As long as you make the right choices, healthy snacking keeps your blood sugars level and increases your energy. Snacking keeps your brain active meaning that you can concentrate and remain focused throughout the day and on into the evening.

If you enjoy your snacks, aim for fruit, plain or unsweetened Greek-style yogurt, celery sticks, carrots or nuts and seeds.

Not Just 5 a Day

We all know that 5 portions of fruit and vegetables a day is the recommended amount. Given the nutritional value in fruit and vegetables and the health benefits of them 5 portions should be your absolute minimum and whilst meal planning you should be looking at ways of increasing your consumption wherever you can.

Try adding fruit to your breakfast cereal or drinking a smoothie instead of a cup of tea for breakfast, be more adventurous with your salads, replace your lunchtime sandwich and crisps with a salad and add vegetables to your pasta sauces, stews and soups and before you know it you will have increased your intake of fruit and veg without even noticing.

Flavour Your Food with Herbs and Spices.

Spices have been found to inhibit the formation of prostaglandins – the hormones that trigger inflammatory reactions. Reduce your use of salt and increase your use of herbs and mild spices to flavour your food instead. Use - cloves, cinnamon, turmeric, rosemary, ginger, sage, and thyme all of which are known for their anti-inflammatory properties.

Scientists in India have found that curcumin, the primary active ingredient of turmeric, has anti – depressant qualities that were found to be at least as effective as certain medications in the treatment of depression – but without the negative side effects.

Refined V Unrefined

Always choose unrefined ingredients over refined ones.

Unrefined foods contain more natural nutrients because they have not been stripped of their vitamins and minerals in the refining process.

Fibre

People who eat a lot of refined foods and skip the fruit and vegetables are missing out on fibre. A lack of fibre in the diet leads to digestive problems and blood sugar imbalances. Fibre is the indigestible portion of grains, vegetables and fruit it is used by the body to improve intestinal function, helps to grow healthy bacteria in the gut and helps prevent disease by removing waste products and toxins from the body. Drop the white bread, pasta and rice and increase fruit, vegetables and whole grains wherever possible.

Eat at least 25 grams of fibre every day. A fibre-rich diet helps reduce inflammation by supplying the body with anti-inflammatory phytonutrients found in fruits, vegetables, and other whole foods. The best sources of fibre are whole grains, such as barley and oatmeal; vegetables such as peas, Brussel sprouts, parsnips and spinach, and fruit such as apples, bananas, oranges, strawberries and raspberries.

Chapter Seven

Top 40 Foods to Include in Your
Anti- Cellulite Food Plan

Apples –

Apples are low in calories and high in fibre. They are full of antioxidants which help flush out toxins from the body as well as containing pectin which is a gel forming fibre that helps to detox the digestive tract, helping to break down cellulite.

Eat more apples: - as well as the obvious, adding an apple to your lunch box each day, apples can be grated onto your morning cereal, grated or sliced into cole slaw, baked on their own with dried fruit and maple syrup, cooked in a pie or juiced.

Apricots –

Apricots are rich in fibre and high in vitamins A and C as well

as containing lycopene which helps to reduce water retention
and stimulate circulation both of which can help fight cellulite.

Eat more apricots: - eat fresh or dry as a snack, add them to
fruit salads, breakfast cereal or yoghurt.

Asparagus –

Asparagus is high in anti-inflammatory properties which are
known to reduce bloating. It is also low in calories making it
perfect for those looking to reduce their weight. Asparagus is
also known to stimulate the bloods circulation which helps to
flush out toxins that can lead to cellulite.

Eat more asparagus: - steam them and eat them on the side,
griddle them, add them to the barbeque, steam them and add
them to salads, quiches and soups.

Bananas –

Bananas are known for being a great energy source as well as
being high in zinc which helps to improve the skin. The
potassium found in bananas helps to boost blood flow which
can help to prevent cellulite.

Eat more bananas: - add them to your cereal, blend them in smoothies add them to yoghurt, milk or fruit salad. Split the skins, wrap them in tin foil and add them to the barbeque – for a little more luxury pour a little brandy into the tin foil before cooking and once cooked serve with cream or ice cream.

Beans –

Aduki beans, borlotti beans, cannelloni beans, Chickpeas, haricot beans, Kidney beans and lentils are high in protein and fibre they contain iron, potassium, magnesium as well as B vitamins.

Beans help to regulate the appetite, lower cholesterol, control blood pressure and help you lose weight which can help to get rid of cellulite. Beans provide a lot of bulk without a lot of calories which fills you up and keeps you satisfied for longer.

Eat more beans: - Make shepherd's pie or lasagna with beans or lentils instead of mince, add them cold to salads, put them in stews and soups. Make pates, hummous and pesto sauce with them.

Bean Sprouts –

Bean sprouts have multiple health benefits, they are not only low in calories but they also contain vitamins A, B, C, D, E and K and essential fatty acids, iron, calcium, magnesium and zinc. These vitamins and minerals help to stimulate blood circulation and aid liver function as well as promoting healthy skin.

Eat more bean sprouts: - add them to salads and stir frys.

Beetroot –

This beautifully coloured root vegetable contains lycopene which helps stimulate circulation as well as reduce water retention. Beetroots also contain potassium which helps boost blood flow, vitamin E which is essential for healthy skin and vitamin A which boosts collagen in the skin.

Eat more beetroot: - juice them with carrots and apples, add the juice to fruit smoothies, bake them in cakes and muffins, eat them roasted, pickled with salads or boiled.

Berries –

Berries are a rich source of toxin fighting antioxidants. Regularly eating raspberries, blackberries, strawberries, cranberries and blueberries is a good way of flushing toxins from the body.

Eat more berries: - sprinkle them on breakfast cereal, add them to yoghurt and smoothies, puddings and baking.

Broccoli –

Broccoli is high in nutritional value. Each floret contains high levels of beauty boosting vitamins and minerals as well as being low in calories.

Broccoli also contains Alpha lipoic which is a naturally occurring substance that prevents collagen from hardening in the body which results in cellulite.

Eat more broccoli: - steam it on the side with a sprinkling of mixed seeds, add it to soups, quiches and stir fries.

Cabbage –

Cabbage is an excellent body cleanser it helps to flush out excess toxins the potassium in cabbage can also relieve water retention.

Eat more cabbage: - shred it into coleslaw, add it to soup, shred it and steam it and mix it into roast potatoes, juice it with celery and apple.

Cayenne Pepper –

Cayenne pepper is believed to boost the metabolism, which helps the body burn more calories as well as helping to improve the body's circulation by increasing blood flow.

Eat more cayenne pepper: - sprinkle it on dips and sauces.

Celery –

Celery, like cucumber is a diuretic food, which can help to relieve water retention and flush out toxins from the body. A build-up of fluid in the body can lead to cellulite.

Eat more celery: - use it as a base in soup, juice it with apple, cucumber and kale, chop it into salads, dip it into hummous, nut butter or fish pate.

Cider Vinegar –

Cider Vinegar is a great detoxifier as it acts as a digestive tonic helping to get rid of harmful bacteria in the intestines, flush out toxins from the body and relieve water retention around the thighs and stomach which helps to reduce the appearance of cellulite.

Eat more cider vinegar: - add it to extra virgin olive oil and pour it over your salad.

Cranberry Juice –

Cranberry Juice like cucumber and celery is a diuretic food which can help flush toxins out of the body and relieve water retention which can lead to cellulite.

Drink more cranberries: - add it to a morning smoothie or just drink it as it is, make sure you only drink sugar free versions.

Cucumber –

Cucumber is a diuretic food, which can help relieve water retention and flush out toxins from the body. A build-up of fluid in the body can trigger the formation of cellulite.

Eat more cucumbers: - chop it into salad, eat it with dips, dice it into tabbouleh, grate it and squeeze out the liquid and add it to plain Greek yoghurt with a little mint seasoning and a splash of lemon juice.

Dandelion –

Dandelion, like nettles, with its diuretic properties is a liver tonic. Dandelion helps rid the body of toxins and flush out excess fluids. Dandelion is a powerful antioxidant, containing vitamins A, C, D and E, zinc, iron and potassium.

Eat more dandelions: - although the leaves are quite bitter they can be added to salads or simply drink it as a tea.

Dong Quai –

Dong Quai regulates the digestive system, reduces bloating and acts as a liver tonic helping it to flush excess toxins from the body which can result in cellulite.

Dong Quai is high in vitamins A, C and E it contains calcium, zinc, magnesium and potassium all of which help fight cellulite.

Eat more Dong Quai: - drink as a tea or take it in capsule form.

Eggs –

Egg yolks are packed with detoxifying vitamins and minerals which can help to flush out excess toxins from the body.

Eat more eggs: - have them poached, boiled, omelet or scrambled, eat them for breakfast, in your packed lunch or in salads.

Fennel –

Fennel aids digestion, reduces inflammation and helps to flush out the excess fluid and toxins that can lead to cellulite. Fennel is also excellent for maintaining healthy hair and skin.

Eat more fennel: - fennel makes a lovely liquorice flavoured tea, shred it into salad or stir fry or roast it either on its own or with other vegetables.

Garlic –

Garlic helps lower cholesterol and boosts the immune system which not only helps to improve the body's overall health but also aids the blood circulation which helps to flush out toxins and fight cellulite.

Eat more garlic: - add crushed or whole cloves to almost anything, salad dressing, vegetables, soups, pizzas, stir fry and stews.

Ginger –

Ginger is known for stimulating the body's circulation. It stimulates the production of digestive enzymes helping the body digest proteins and fats more fully. Ginger also increases the body's metabolic rate helping it to burn more calories.

Eat more ginger: - add it to curries, stir fry and baking or drink it as a tea.

Grapefruit –

Pink Grapefruit, like watermelon contains the potent antioxidant lycopene which helps to improve blood circulation and smooth out cellulite. Grapefruits, like oranges also contain methoxylated bioflavonoids which help to correct cell imbalances that can lead to cellulite. Grapefruit also boosts the metabolism which aids weight loss.

Eat more grapefruit: - Eat it fresh for breakfast, add tinned (not in syrup) or fresh segments to salad or drink it as a juice.

Green Tea –

Green tea is understood to speed up the body's metabolism, inhibit fat absorption and help regulate the body's glucose levels all of which aid weight loss.

Green tea contains theobromine which is known to stimulate the release the body's stored fat.

Drink more green tea: - drink it morning, noon and night, try swapping at least one if not more or your daily cups of tea for a green cup. Try mint green tea for a change.

Lemons –

Lemons can aid the rebalancing of the body's acid-alkali keeping it at a steady PH, meaning that your body is better able to support healthy bacteria and assist the removal of toxins which can lead to cellulite.

Eat more lemons: - add lemon juice to salad dressings.

Live Bio Yoghurt –

Live bio yoghurt is full of probiotics and in terms of aiding weight loss it is considered a superfood. Yoghurt is now known to have a significant impact on eliminating fat from the body and that includes cellulite.

Eat more live bio yoghurt: - eat it for breakfast with fruit and a sprinkling of chopped nuts or mixed seeds. Add it to sauces or have it on the side of salads or curries.

Mango –

Mangos are packet with vitamins C and E as well as potassium. Mangos also contain beta-carotene which promotes healthy new cells and boosts the natural elasticity of the skin, creating smoother more evenly textured skin even in cellulite affected areas. The vitamin C in mangos helps to strengthen collagen in the skin.

Eat more mangos: - Eat them fresh or dried as a snack, add them to cereal, smoothies or fruit salads.

Nettles –

Nettles are packed with antioxidants. Their diuretic properties help to eliminate the toxins that cause cellulite and relieve water retention.

Eat more nettles: - nettles should be picked in early spring whilst the plant is young. In late spring use only the tips and young leaves. Wear rubber gloves when collecting to prevent being stung, the sting decreases as the plant is cooked or dried. Add nettles to soups and pesto omelette or steamed greens or drink as a tea.

Nuts –

Walnuts, almonds, brazils, cashews, hazelnuts, macadamia, peanuts, pine nuts, pistachios and walnuts are all high sources of fibre, and protein. They contain vitamins B and E, potassium and magnesium.

Snacking on nuts will help curb hunger, feed your skin and lower your cholesterol and help control blood pressure. Nuts help you lose weight.

Eat more nuts: - Eat a handful of mixed nuts as a snack, sprinkle chopped nuts onto yoghurt, cereal and salad, add them to your morning smoothie. Nut butters can be eaten with dried fruit, added to baking or spread on toast, try nut milks as an alternative to cow milk.

Oily Fish –

Oily fish contain "good fats". Good fats contain fatty acids which can help the body to metabolise fat including cellulite fat.

Avoid "bad fats" found in processed foods such as biscuits, pastries, cheese and sausages. These fats cause cellulite.

Eat more oily fish: - Mackerel, salmon, sardines and tuna are
the most obvious choices. Try to eat 2 / 3 servings a week.
Eat fish poached, baked or grilled, cook them on the
barbeque, make fish pie or fish pate, flake them into salad.

Oranges –

Oranges are packed with vitamin C. Vitamin C prevents
inflammation and strengthens the collagen in your skin.
Strengthened collagen helps to smooth the appearance of
cellulite and reducing inflammation will lessen the excess
weight around a cellulite prone area, in turn decreasing the
severity of cellulite. Oranges also contain methoxylated
bioflavonoids which help improve the blood circulation and
correct imbalances in cells that may lead to cellulite.

Eat more oranges: - Eat them fresh, add segments to salad
or drink them as juice.

Rose Hips –

Rose hips can be made into a syrup and drunk as a winter
tonic or drunk as a tea. Rose hips have been recognised for
their qualities for centuries, in herbal lore the rose is believed
to be good for the skin and soul. Amongst rose hips many
health benefits they aid blood circulation, flush out excess
toxins and hydrate the skin.

Eat more rose hips: - Drink it as tea or make a syrup or cordial.

Rosemary –

Rosemary is believed to improve the body's digestion of fats keeping wastes from building up, including cellulite deposits.

Eat more rosemary: - Add it to roasted vegetables or drink it in tea.

Seeds –

Flaxseeds, sesame seeds, pumpkin seeds and the oil derived from them are all good sources of vitamin E which is essential for healthy skin and magnesium, iron protein and fibre. Seeds help maintain healthy skin, regulate your appetite and lower your cholesterol. Seeds are high in protein and healthy fats, they have one of the lowers GI values of all foods, which means that they help maintain steady blood sugar levels which results in balanced energy levels with minimal fat storage.

Eat more seeds: - Like nuts, sprinkle over cereal, yoghurt, salad, stews and soups.

Spinach –

Low calorie spinach will not only help you improve your skin, but it will also help you lose weight. Spinach is high in vitamin A, which aids the production of collagen in the skin helping to reduce the appearance of cellulite. Collagen is a protein that helps to strengthen, smooth and plump up the skin.

Eat more spinach: - Eat it fresh in salad, or cooked as a vegetable. Make pesto with it, put it in an omelette, add it to potatoes for a pie filling or blend it in your morning smoothie.

Tomatoes –

Tomatoes vibrant red colour comes from lycopene which stimulates the circulatory system and reduces fluid retention. Tomatoes are also rich in vitamin C which helps to keep the skin firm and tout by aiding the production of collagen.

Eat more tomatoes: - add it to salads, sandwiches and pizza, stews and soup.

Turmeric –

Like Cayenne pepper, turmeric can help getting rid of cellulite. Turmeric is known for its high levels of antioxidants, it stimulates the circulation, reduces swelling and helps to flush out toxins from the body.

Eat more turmeric: - add it to a low-calorie curry or stir it into rice or grains.

Water –

One of the most common causes of cellulite is a build-up of toxins in the body. Toxins slow down the body's circulation which can lead to cellulite, they also reduce the skins elasticity which makes the cellulite appear more obvious.

Water aids the body's natural detox process and helps to flush unwanted toxins out.

Drink more water: - try to drink the recommended daily amount of 8 glasses, this includes tea, herbal tea and sugar free cordial. Drink more if the weather is hot or you have been exercising.

Watermelon –

Watermelon contains the antioxidant lycopene which is where it gets its wonderful colour from. Lycopene helps to improve blood circulation which can over time help to smooth out cellulite.

Eat more watermelon: - Eat it fresh cut into segments, cube it and add it to fruit salad or blend it in your morning smoothie.

Wholegrains –

Whole grain cereals, oats, rye, barley, wheat, buckwheat, quinoa, millet and brown rice are all a source of slow release energy helping us to feel fuller for longer. Whole grains keep the body's blood sugar levels balanced, preventing energy spikes which lead to cravings for sugary foods – sugary foods cause cellulite.

Whole grains are also high in antioxidants which help the body to flush out toxins which can lead to cellulite.

Eat more wholegrains: - Look for whole grain alternatives to the normal white bread, pasta and rice. Eat more porridge, muesli and wholegrain cereals. Add cooked grains to salads, stews and soups.

Chapter Eight

Vitamins and Minerals that Help Fight Cellulite.

Vitamin A

Vitamin A is a powerful antioxidant that helps your skin repair collagen and connective tissues. Uneven connective tissues are a cause of the lumpy appearance of cellulite. Vitamin A also fights toxins, preventing future cellulite damage. Vitamin A sources include potato, mango, spinach and carrots or it can be taken as a supplement.

Vitamin B6

Vitamin B6 helps your body metabolise nutrients that increase your skin's elasticity. It also helps rid your body of excess liquid that can make the appearance of cellulite more severe. Increasing your intake of vitamin B6 can, over time help fight the appearance of cellulite. Vitamin B6 is found in whole grains, vegetables, bananas and nuts or can be taken as a supplement.

Vitamin C

Vitamin C prevents inflammation and strengthens the collagen in your skin, which helps to smooth the appearance of cellulite. Decreasing inflammation lessens the excess weight around a cellulite prone area. Good sources of vitamin C include strawberries, oranges, broccoli, red pepper, lemon and Brussels sprouts or it can be taken as a supplement.

Vitamin E

Vitamin E improves circulation and increases your skin's elasticity by increasing the production of collagen. Improved elasticity helps to smooth the fatty lumps created by cellulite and decreases its appearance. Increasing your intake of vitamin E, will help reduce cellulite. Vitamin E sources include sweet potato, pumpkin, nuts, seeds, papaya, broccoli and tomatoes or it can be taken as a supplement.

Lycopene

Lycopene gives certain fruit and vegetables their bright colours. Lycopene improves blood circulation and helps flush excess toxins from the body. Good sources of lycopene are watermelon, tomatoes, berries, apricots and beetroot.

Methoxylated bioflavonoids

Methoxylated bioflavonoids help the blood circulate and correct any imbalances in the cells that lead to cellulite. Good sources are oranges and grapefruit.

Potassium

Potassium helps boost blood flow and relieve water retention which in turn helps get rid of cellulite and prevent it from forming in the future. Good sources of potassium are bananas, beetroot, mango, dandelion, cabbage and nuts.

Words of Encouragement.

Our diet is the key to our happiness, we can literally change anything through our diet.

- Eat more fruit and veg ▪Dump the junk, ▪ Take up an activity

- Don't wait for tomorrow – start today.

It really is that simple.

While the author has made every effort to ensure that the information contained in this book is as accurate and up to date as possible, it is advisory only and should not be used as an alternative to seeking specialist medical advice. The author cannot be held responsible for actions that may be taken by the reader as a result of reliance on the information contained in this book, which are taken entirely at the readers own risk.

©2018 Laura Hails

Laura Hails asserts the moral right to be identified as the author of this work. All rights reserved. No part of this publication may be reproduced, stored in a retrieval system, or transmitted in any form or by any means, electrical, mechanical, photocopying, recording or otherwise, without the prior written permission of the author.

.